CELEBRATE NURSING

HUMAN BY BIRTH—HERO BY CHOICE

Renee Thompson, DNP, RN, CMSRN

Joanne Turka, MSN, RN-BC, Alumnus CCRN

Disclaimer: This book is not intended as medical, career, or legal advice.

To contact the authors, visit www.RTConnections.com

To contact the publisher, inCredible Messages Press, visit www.inCredibleMessages.com

Printed in the United States of America

ISBN 978-0-9889266-4-6   Paperback

-Inspirational   -Personal Growth

Book Shepherd / Coaching ....: Bonnie Budzowski, inCredible Messages, LP
Interior Design ....: inCredible Messages, LP
Cover Design ....: Bobbie Fox, Bobbie Fox, Inc.

To protect confidentiality, names and some details of the stories in this book have been changed.

DEDICATION

This book is for you and all other nurses, current and future. As a nurse, you perform heroic acts every day, even if you don't yet view yourself as a hero. Believe that you make a difference—because you do!

The strongest principle of growth lies in human choice.

—George Eliot

CONTENTS

Introduction 1

Hero Nurse... 3

Extend Compassion 4

Communicate with Openness and Respect 14

Build Relationships 26

Develop Hardiness.. 36

Keep Learning.. 46

Laugh.. 54

Live with Integrity 62

Think Positive.. 70

Own Your Practice 80

Strengthen Moral Courage 88

So What, Now What?..................................... 98

About the Authors... 100

Book Renee Thompson for Your Next Event 107

INTRODUCTION

CHANCES ARE THAT NURSES, as a group, are the most compassionate people in the world. In fact, most of us enter the profession because we want to make a difference. We want to give patients the best and most compassionate care so they can heal.

Unfortunately, with heavy workloads, stressful environments, and constant changes in technology, it's easy to lose the focus that motivated us to become nurses. It can be a struggle simply to come to work each day. Yet, in the face of all this, some nurses rise to the level of hero. They stand out from the rest in their ability to provide extraordinary care in the midst of constant stress and demand. How do they do it?

Every nurse has the opportunity to be a hero, every day. Heroes aren't magic nurses who have abilities the rest of us simply don't have. Every nurse engages in hero behaviors. Engaging in these behaviors *consistently* allows a nurse to rise to the top and have the greatest possible positive influence.

Being a hero doesn't mean you have to travel across the globe to open an orphanage. You are a hero to a patient when you call the physician at home at 2 o'clock in the morning to get adequate pain medication, despite the repercussions. You are a hero to a new nurse when you go out of your way to help her manage her first patient crisis. You are a hero to a family when you comfort a husband whose wife was just diagnosed with terminal cancer even though you don't have the time.

In this book you will explore ten hero powers—behaviors that distinguish hero nurses from the rest. You'll read heartwarming stories of real nurses who demonstrate each behavior. These nurses truly represent the art and science of nursing and are role models for others. We are confident you can be a role model too.

This book is meant to provide inspiration and practical tips to help you become more heroic in your practice and to inspire you to believe you make a difference.

Being a hero is a choice.

There are 3.1 million practicing nurses in this country and close to 200,000 aspiring nurses in nursing schools. Just imagine the positive impact nurses can make by choosing to be heroes.

It all begins with you.

Choose to make a difference—choose to be a hero!

HERO NURSE

DEFINITION:

he•ro

A nurse who consistently engages in a cluster of behaviors that combine to provide exceptional care to patients and their families.

Here are the ten behaviors of hero nurses:

- Extend compassion
- Communicate with openness and respect
- Build relationships
- Develop hardiness
- Keep learning
- Laugh
- Live with integrity
- Think positively
- Own your practice
- Strengthen moral courage

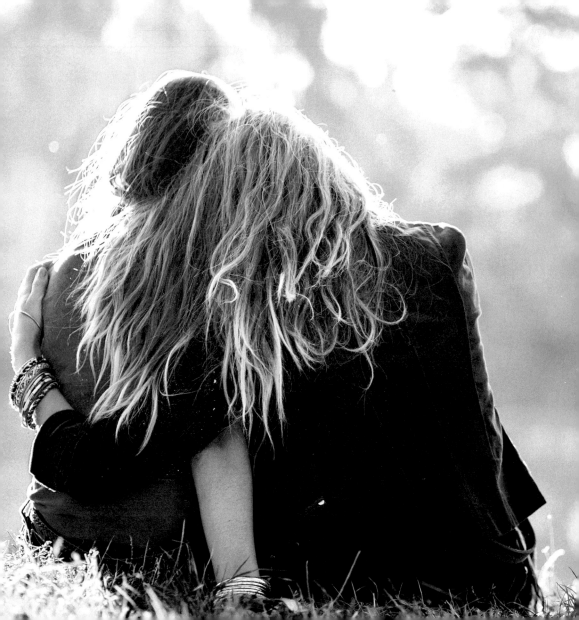

> *Be kind, for every-one you meet is fighting a hard battle.*
>
> *—Plato*

EXTEND COMPASSION

AMY, A STAFF NURSE IN THE NEONATAL ICU, watched Jason stare down at his new daughter. Jason's shock and confusion were obvious as he looked at tiny Charlotte. Jason would be unable to hold Charlotte for another 24 hours. She was too fragile, and the life-saving wires and tubes supporting her were in the way.

Gradually, Amy learned the heartbreaking story of this family. Jason and his wife, Jess, had been so excited about the birth of their third daughter. Jason said Jess was like a broken record throughout the pregnancy, saying, "I just can't wait to see and hold Charlotte."

At 38 weeks, on a beautiful summer day, Jess and Jason made the trek to the hospital for the induced labor. Two hours into labor, Jess began to have trouble breathing. She turned to her left side to move the baby a bit and experienced a cardiac arrest from an anaphylactic response from an amniotic fluid embolism.

Chaos ensued; Charlotte was delivered emergently by cesarean section, intubated, and transferred to the Neonatal Intensive Care Unit (NICU). Jess was also intubated and transferred to the Medical Intensive Care Unit (MICU).

During the next 48 hours, Jess hemorrhaged and struggled to live while Charlotte remained in the NICU.

Jason, surrounded by family and friends, was stunned. He told anyone who would listen that Jess just wanted to see and hold her new baby. Unfortunately, the baby wasn't stable enough to leave the NICU, and Jess wasn't stable enough to leave the MICU.

Amy observed how Jason visited Charlotte, unable to hold her at first. As soon as possible, Amy adjusted the life-saving wires and tubes so Charlotte's two big sisters could see their new sister without being scared. As the baby became more stable, Amy provided Jason with a rocking chair and support to allow him to hold, feed, and talk to Charlotte. Amy listened as

Jason repeatedly related that Jess just wanted to see and hold her baby.

Three days passed. News from the MICU got worse and worse. Jess had two strokes and was in a coma. She had acute kidney injury and now required daily dialysis. Jess might never wake up.

The nurses, especially Amy, observed as Jason traveled many times a day from the MICU (reading to Jess and telling her about their beautiful new baby), to the NICU (feeding and caring for the baby).

Eventually, Charlotte became stable enough to be discharged to go home without her mom. That's when Amy began to extend remarkable acts of compassion.

Contacting the physician team and hospital administration, Amy arranged for Charlotte to remain a patient in the hospital for two additional days to make it easier for Jason to visit both his wife and infant daughter. Family and friends were caring for the two older children.

The following day, Amy reported off in the NICU. Amy then visited Jason in the MICU. She asked if Jason would like her to bring Charlotte (now medically stable) to him at Jess's bedside.

Jason, exhausted, agreed. He continued to read and talk to Jess. A few hours later, Amy wheeled Charlotte into the MICU in her tiny enclosed bed, complete with bottles, diapers, and other care items.

Even though invasive lines, drainage tubes, dialysis machines, and EEG machines made close contact difficult, Amy intuitively knew mom and baby should have skin-to-skin contact.

With Jason's consent, Amy un-swaddled Charlotte and placed her on Jess's unconscious body. Amy physically moved Jess's left arm to the "baby holding" position and ensured both baby and mommy were safe. Jason and Amy watched as Charlotte immediately snuggled into her mommy's unconscious body. Would Jess respond in any way?

A single tear streamed from Jess's right eye—there was no other visible neurologic response. That single tear was enough for Jason; he was overwhelmed with emotion and hope. A single act of compassion by an amazing, astute nurse had provided Jason with a sign that his wife might have some brain function and might survive.

The recovery continued over months and years as Jess regained consciousness, experienced intensive rehabilitation, and returned to the role of functioning wife and mother, with some minor stroke deficits (for details, go to www.inspired-recovery.net).

DEFINITION:
com•pas•sion
> Compassion is sympathetic concern for the sufferings of others, coupled with a desire to alleviate it. When nurses show genuine concern for patients, and then do everything they can to comfort them, their hero powers rise.

Amy demonstrated a hero's dose of compassion in many ways. She provided exceptional care to Jason and the two "big sisters," beginning in the NICU when she converted the tube-intensive environment into a welcoming place to care for and nurture this new baby.

Amy identified Jason's need to be at the sides of both his wife and daughter. She intervened by encouraging and assisting physicians and administrators to create a plan to extend Charlotte's hospital stay by several days. After leaving work, Amy used her personal time to perform a powerful compassionate act: allowing an unconscious mother to "hold" her new baby.

Tips to Develop and Improve Compassion

Practice Daily Acts of Kindness

Acts of kindness to others generate a feeling of happiness and satisfaction in you. Throughout the course of your ordinary days, look for simple ways to extend kindness to family members, colleagues, and friends. Acknowledge the difficulties and stresses those around you face.

Reach Out to Strangers

It is often most rewarding to extend your kindness to a stranger. For example, one physician has a daily routine in his hospital cafeteria. He pays for the meal of the person behind him in the checkout line.

The checkout personnel know the doctor's routine and perform the transaction without a word. This act costs the physician between five and eight dollars a day. The gratification for both the physician and the "next guest" is worth far more than that. Most acts of kindness cost nothing: opening a door, picking up a dropped item, smiling at a stranger.

PRACTICE DAILY REFLECTION

Once a day, reflect on the 24 hours you just had. Consciously think about what made the day good or bad. Especially think about your own actions. What did you do to influence the overall tone of the day, for better or worse? If it was a great day, think about which of your actions contributed to make the day great. Then try to repeat those actions and think of all the great days in store for you!

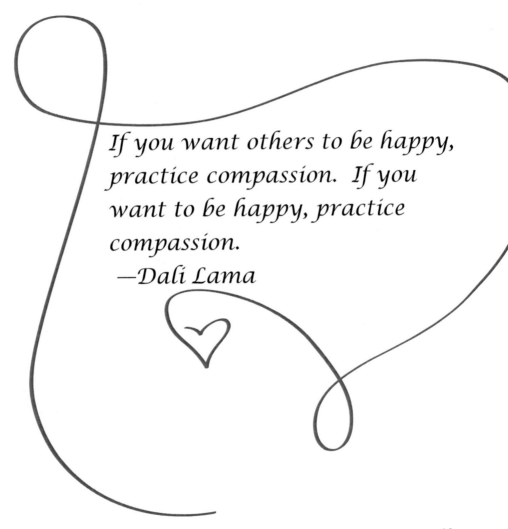

If you want others to be happy,
practice compassion. If you
want to be happy, practice
compassion.
  —Dali Lama

The basic building block of good communications is the feeling that every human being is unique and of value.
— *Unknown*

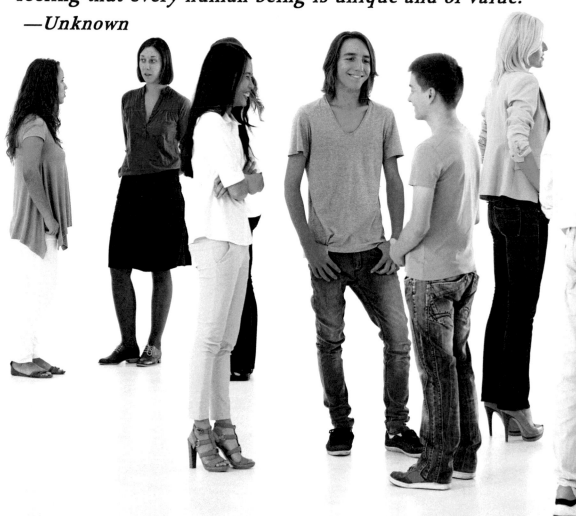

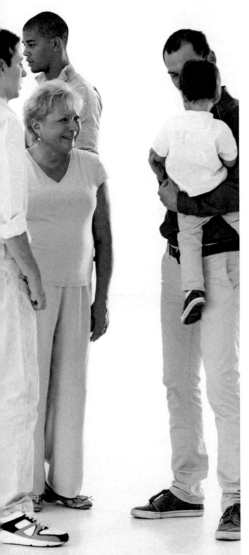

COMMUNICATE WITH OPENNESS AND RESPECT

RED-VESTED TRIBAL LEADERS and a communication gap the size of the Grand Canyon stood between Perry and his team as they cared for their patient, Mrs. Two Moons.

The matriarch of a large Montana American Indian tribe, Mrs. Two Moons, age 76, was known as Mother or Aunt to literally dozens of tribal members, from small children to weathered adults. One day, Mrs. Two Moons suffered a massive cerebral vascular accident and landed in the care of Perry and his team in the ICU. When Perry first met Mrs. Two Moons, she was comatose, and the medical staff was working hard to keep her alive.

Over the next few hours, dozens of Mrs. Two Moons' family, friends, and tribal members poured into the hospital. The ICU waiting room became Mrs. Two Moons' waiting room. The phones and door buzzer were soon overwhelmed with calls and requests to see Mrs. Two Moons. Many of the tribal members traveled over 100 miles to the hospital without food, extra clothes, money, or a place to stay.

As Mrs. Two Moons fought for her life, Perry divided his time between talking with Mrs. Two Moons' distraught family and friends and listening to his frustrated staff members. While Mrs. Two Moons' support gathered, Perry gathered his own support team. He called the chaplain and social worker to help him calm the crowd. For a few days, they were able to manage the situation. Then one day, the tribal leader, a large American Indian, asked to speak to Perry alone. Frankly, Perry felt intimidated.

The tribal leader explained that in his tribe, Mrs. Two Moons was considered his aunt although not by blood. He said, "She is a member of my family and we are here to honor her." The tribal leader demanded a meeting with senior hospital officials and Perry at 8:00 a.m. the next morning. While Perry didn't know how he was going to manage to pull a high-level meeting together on such short notice, he didn't have the courage to refuse.

The following morning, six large and imposing men wearing red vests were waiting for Perry when he came in the door. Walking to the conference room, the atmosphere was tense, with little eye contact between tribal members and hospital staff. The men refused the customary coffee and rolls.

The meeting commenced, with the red-vested tribal leaders on one side of the table and the white-coated hospital leaders on the other. The tribal leader stood and said, "Do you see these red vests we are wearing? These are our ceremonial battle garments. We are here to do battle for our aunt and mother. We are here to demand our rights."

"We insist that our shaman (medicine man) be allowed to spend time with Mrs. Two Moons, and we demand that others get a chance to see her as well. We also insist that the shaman be permitted to place soil in her bed and burn some sweet grass in the room. The smoke must come in contact with her."

The room grew silent. Hospital staff members were thinking, "We have rules in our hospital, strict visiting hours and limitations on who can stay and for how long. For goodness sake, we can't let someone put dirt in a critically ill patient's bed and light a fire in her room. What would the Joint Commission say about that?"

As the silence continued, the communication gap felt wider and wider. Perry felt like the two sides were speaking different languages. Then he had a moment of clarity. Perry realized he understood these tribal members' language: they were advocating for their aunt. They wore their red vests to communicate they were willing to fight to protect their family member, just as Perry would fight for his.

Perry realized that everyone wanted the same thing: for Mrs. Two Moons to get the best care possible. The two groups simply had different ways of understanding the path forward. In that moment, Perry understood that he needed to communicate in a way that was respectful and kind, yet assertive, while considering the needs of the hospital as well as American Indian culture.

Perry stood, took a deep breath, and spoke, using his best soothing but professional voice. He thanked the tribal members for sharing their needs, vowing to do everything possible to ensure their aunt was taken care of according to their wishes. With this assurance, both sides were able to work collaboratively toward a solution.

Hospital leaders agreed to allow the shaman into the room and to place a small amount of soil near the feet of Mrs. Two Moons. They also allowed a small amulet containing a feather, some soil, and some different types of plants into the bed. As the ICU was on the first floor of the hospital, they agreed to move Mrs. Two Moons' bed near the window. The shaman would burn the sweet grass outside her window, and the smoke would come in from the outside and contact her.

Perry explained the strategy to his staff, who were at first hesitant and even angry. "We just can't let these people tell us how to care for our patients," said one irate staff member. Perry used the opportunity to help his staff see how important it was to communicate openly and respectfully with the tribal members and to listen with their hearts as well as their heads.

The shaman arrived, waved the smoke over Mrs. Two Moons' body, placed some objects in her bed, talked, sang, and prayed. The experience was beautiful, and Perry felt honored to be in the room at the time. The ceremony was focused, sincere, and directed as treatment for Mrs. Two Moons. At that point, the shaman became part of the ICU team. After the event, the shaman explained parts of the ceremony and their importance.

While Mrs. Two Moons passed away, she did so in a peaceful atmosphere that honored her deeply held beliefs. What started as a complicated and adversarial event ended as a death with dignity, in the presence of loved ones, and respectful of tribal customs. The tribal leader shook Perry's hand and thanked him for working to bring the two sides together and for his willingness to listen.

Definition:

com•mu•ni•cate

> Almost 200,000 people die each year from the effects of adverse medical events. Eighty five percent of those deaths can be somehow linked to poor communication. Nurses who articulate honestly, assertively, and respectfully save lives.

In his experience with Mrs. Two Moons, Perry demonstrated the hero behavior of effective communication. He actively listened until he understood the motive behind the seeming belligerent demands of Mrs. Two Moons' advocates. Once he understood, Perry was able to offer respect and flexibility to the tribe, without compromising the hospital's patient safety standards. He demonstrated how to advocate for humans, as individuals, to his staff and other healthcare professionals.

Tips for Open and Respectful Communication

> *You can make more friends in two weeks by becoming a good listener than you can in two years trying to get other people interested in you.*
> —Dale Carnegie

Actively Listen

The manner in which you listen is often more important than what you say. Follow these simple dos and don'ts to improve your ability to listen:

Do maintain eye contact with the person who is speaking

Do offer affirmation and acknowledgment

Don't interrupt

Don't rehearse in your head what you plan to say next

SPEAK ASSERTIVELY

Assertive communicators are respectful active listeners; they are considerate of others and honest (no games). They also insist upon respect for their own viewpoints and standards. To speak more assertively, start conversations using phrases like the following:

"Help me to understand . . . ."

"I'm concerned about . . . ."

"I'm not sure you realize this but . . . ."

"How can we resolve this?"

"I feel strongly about this because . . . ."

"While I am willing to be flexible, I am unwilling to compromise patient safety."

PAUSE BEFORE YOU SPEAK

Pausing allows you to gather your thoughts, to consider the situation, the people involved, and the potential outcomes. It allows you to take the time you need to formulate a good response. Use the pause when you receive an inflammatory e-mail, before you get involved in a conflict situation, or when you have to address bad behavior or bad practice.

Speak Up

Less than 10% of nurses speak up when witnessing bad behavior or bad practice. Why? Many nurses are afraid of retaliation or fear how the other person will respond. Some just don't have the skill set to address situations involving conflict. However, nurses have an ethical responsibility to the public to speak up when they witness behavior that could compromise patient outcomes.

When you witness bad behavior or bad practice, ask yourself, "Does this behavior have the potential to negatively impact patient care?" If the answer is, "Yes," speak up assertively and respectfully.

Be Curious about Differences

The root of many misconceptions and conflicts is simple misunderstanding. When a co-worker or patient is different from you (race, ethnicity, culture, and gender are only the obvious ones), ask sincere questions. Demonstrate curiosity and respect. Look for things in common as points of connection. Celebrate healthy differences. Express your desire to honor values and traditions different from your own.

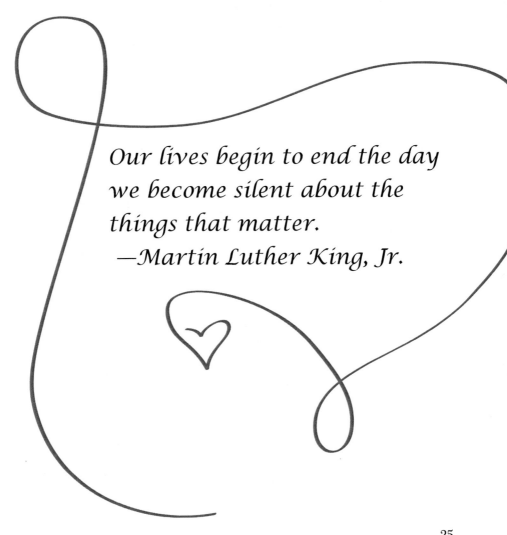

Our lives begin to end the day
we become silent about the
things that matter.
—Martin Luther King, Jr.

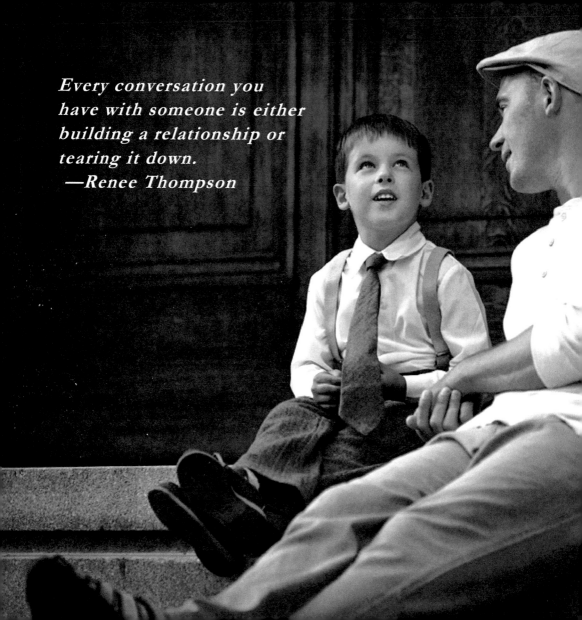

Every conversation you have with someone is either building a relationship or tearing it down.
—Renee Thompson

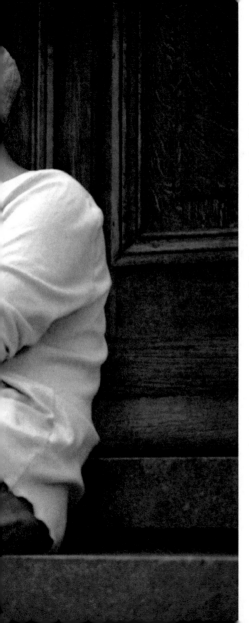

BUILD RELATIONSHIPS

WALKING INTO WORK THAT DAY, Danielle was apprehensive. In fact, every day Danielle came to work, she was a bit apprehensive. After eight years off the hospital floor, she recently returned to bedside nursing, working casual on a trauma step-down unit. While Danielle had spent the last 10 years in a doctor's office, there's nothing like the challenge of a hospital unit.

The clinical environment is so complex now that even with two decades worth of experience, Danielle felt like an amateur nurse again. Each workday provided another learning challenge. In addition, Danielle was acutely aware of the deep-seated culture of bullying in healthcare. Any-

27

body with a fresh-scrubbed look or many questions is a prime target.

Walking onto her unit that day, Danielle felt the apprehension like butterflies in her left side. She wondered, "What type of assignment will I have? With whom will I be working? Will I be able to handle today's patients?" It had been three months since Danielle started her casual job, and still these thoughts troubled her as she walk into work.

Danielle didn't see her name on the assignment sheet for the day. Then the charge nurse said something that shook Danielle to her core, "Oh. You got pulled to another unit."

"WHAT?" she thought. "I am barely able to keep up with my responsibilities on my unit let alone on a different unit."

Danielle took a deep breath, put on her best fake confidence face, and walked the "green mile" to the short stay unit. On the way, she thought about what typically happens to agency, float pool, and travel nurses: They get the worst assignments, are targets of bullies, and suffer the brunt of EVERYBODY'S bad mood. Danielle braced herself as she walked onto the unit.

The first person Danielle met was the night nurse, Kathy, who greeted her with a smile and asked, "Are you Danielle?"

When she nodded affirmatively, Kathy smiled and said, "Welcome." Then Kathy shouted, "Hey Kara, Danielle is here."

Kara, the charge nurse, came out of the break room wearing a smile and said something the nervous nurse would never forget, "You're going to love it here today. We're going to do everything we can to make sure you have a great day."

As the nurses and unit secretary smiled and welcomed Danielle, she was stunned. This isn't how things go for floating nurses on the hospital unit. Danielle felt as if she had walked onto a healthcare unit in an alternate universe—one where it is safe to concentrate on patients rather than protecting yourself from your co-workers. Danielle took her first breath since leaving her home unit. It was going to be okay.

What started as potentially the worst day turned into the best day Danielle had had since returning to clinical practice. Ruth, the nurse who gave Danielle report, went out of her way to make sure she set Danielle up to succeed. She got Danielle's med cart set up, stocked it with everything needed, put extra bags of IV fluid in each patient's room, and told Danielle specifically whom to call if she needed anything for each patient. Throughout the day, Kara, the charge nurse, checked in with

Danielle, asking if she needed anything. Danielle never felt like a novice or a bother, even as she tortured Kara with questions.

In the afternoon, just as Danielle was feeling settled and confident, she learned she was getting an admission. Ugh. The stress level shot back up.

While taking care of her other patient, Danielle's admission came. When she finally had the chance to ask about her admission, Danielle discovered that Rachel, another nurse on the unit, had already settled Danielle's new patient, checked vital signs, hooked her up to the monitor, and let the physicians know the patient was there. Really? Yes.

Whenever someone came to the unit, Kara greeted that person with a smile: physicians, patients' family members, respiratory therapists, pharmacy technicians, dietary and housekeepers, everyone. It made no difference what role the visitor had. Each person was treated with kindness and respect.

On the unit that day, it was easy for Danielle to see that Kara's commitment to positive relationships infuses her whole unit. The nurses who work on Kara's unit extend the respect and kindness they receive from Kara to others.

DEFINITION:
re•la•tion•ship

> The success of any organization depends on its ability to build and sustain meaningful relationships with employees and customers. In healthcare, building relationships can be a matter of life and death. Nurses are the common link that connects all members of the healthcare team into one. When nurses build positive relationships with others, on or off their own unit, their hero powers soar.

Kara's relationship-building behavior makes her a hero who creates a culture of collaboration as well as competence. Everyone benefits from the way this group behaves.

While not all nurses can be charge nurses, every nurse has a sphere of influence. All nurses make continual choices about how cooperative and collaborative they will be. Nurses who have good relationships with physicians, other nurses, and support staff are able to provide effective care to patients, avoid mistakes, and increase the satisfaction of patients under their care.

Tips to Build Relationships

> *It is one of the most beautiful compensations of this life that no man can sincerely try to help another without helping himself.*
> —*Ralph Waldo Emerson*

Express Gratitude to the People around You

Thank the nursing assistant for bathing your patient. Thank the physical therapist for walking your patient or getting him or her out of bed. When expressing thanks, be specific rather than general.

Pitch In

When possible, help your co-workers. Let the physical therapist know if he or she needs an extra hand getting a patient out of bed, you are available—even if the patient isn't yours. Surprise a nursing assistant by offering to help bathe a patient. Take time to be kind to anyone new on the unit, regardless of that person's discipline. Not only does kindness smooth the day for all involved, it builds relationships in priceless ways.

CELEBRATE SUCCESSES

Find opportunities to celebrate everything good about your co-workers: birthdays, degrees, awards, promotions—everything. Celebrating can involve giving a simple card, ordering out for pizza, bringing in a cake, or publicly recognizing accomplishments.

BE WILLING TO APOLOGIZE

The most powerful three-word phrase in the English language is, "I am sorry." When you admit your mistakes and apologize, you knock down barriers that might be preventing relationships from developing.

INITIATE SUPPORTIVE CONVERSATIONS

Examples include the following:

To new nurse: "I'm going to do everything I can to help you succeed."

To student nurse: "I'm so glad you're here. I will do everything I can to help you learn."

To nursing assistant: "Let's work together today to care for our patients. I can't do it without you."

To therapist: "Please let me know what I can do to support your efforts today."

To patient: "What can I do to make your stay here more comfortable?"

To patient's family member: "I know this must be a difficult time for you. Is there anything I can do for you?"

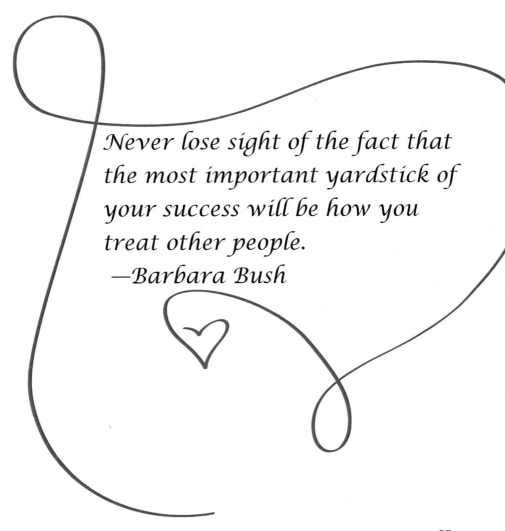

Never lose sight of the fact that the most important yardstick of your success will be how you treat other people.

—Barbara Bush

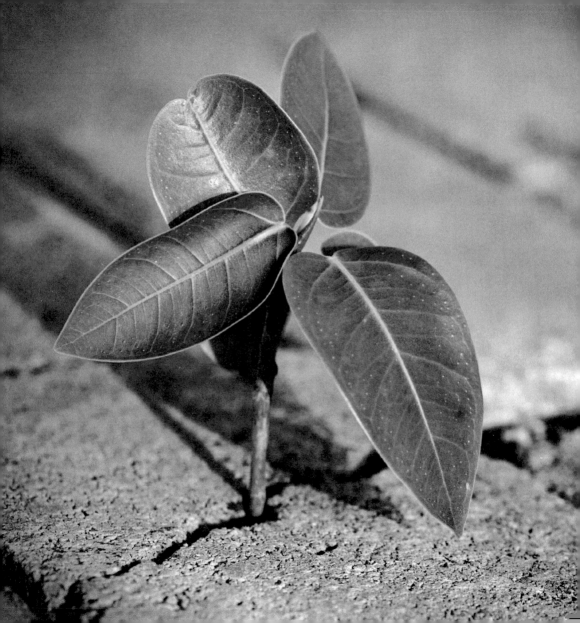

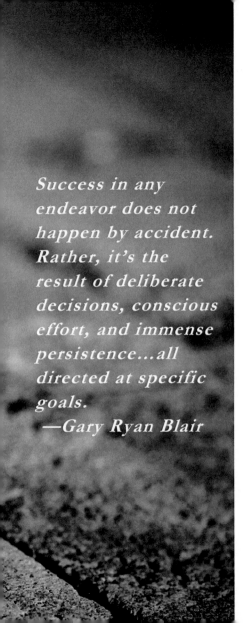

Success in any endeavor does not happen by accident. Rather, it's the result of deliberate decisions, conscious effort, and immense persistence…all directed at specific goals.
—*Gary Ryan Blair*

DEVELOP HARDINESS

A CUP OF JAVA IN HER HAND, Sandy studied the assignment board in the delivery suite. Several moms were being induced that day. Noticing that one delivery would be special, Sandy took a deep breath. The mom was carrying a male baby with trisomy 13.

The trisomy 13 chromosome defect can result in a baby born with a multiple issues: cleft lip and palate, missing eyes, extra or missing digits, and brain and other organ dysfunction. A male baby with trisomy 13 has a life expectancy of roughly 5-10 hours. To make things more challenging, Sandy was assigned to orient a new nurse to the labor and delivery department that day.

With 12 years of obstetric and delivery experience, Sandy selected a room in the rear of the department for this difficult event. In choosing a room far from the other rooms, Sandy hoped to spare the couple from hearing the cries of healthy babies. Sandy taped a single green leaf on the door of the room. A single green leaf is the code to alert all disciplines of a difficult, possibly tragic, delivery. In addition to guiding the new nurse through the setup of the room, Sandy prepared her for the day and the arrival of the expectant parents.

Promptly at 7:30 a.m., the expectant parents arrived. The young, well-educated couple presented Sandy with a complete typewritten list of their choices for the birth and advanced directives for the care of their newborn son. These choices included an immediate baptism by the nursing staff or a pastor, and a request that Dad get to hold their son right after the baptism.

The parents knew the baby may not survive long, and they wanted to make the most of every moment. Another family member, a grandmother, who happened to also be a nurse, was in the waiting room, expecting to be present for the delivery. The typewritten list of expectations, as well as the additional family member, added intensity to the challenging day.

Sandy welcomed the parents to the delivery area and set up the room for their comfort. Mom was attached to all of the electronic monitoring devices and the grandmother was brought into the room. Sandy helped the new nurse with the equipment, explaining everything she was doing. She was supportive and honest in all her interactions.

The room was full of the life-and-death tension of this situation, but Sandy attended to every detail of the patient's requests. Sandy supported the patient, husband, and grandmother throughout the exhausting labor experience. As she monitored this family, she also directed the new nurse's actions and made sure the new nurse understood all the processes that are involved in a difficult labor and delivery.

By 3:00 p.m., the physician was in place, and the labor room was transformed into a delivery suite. Sandy orchestrated personnel in and out of the room as the birth became imminent.

Baby Evan was born. His color dusky blue, Evan had both a cleft lip and palate, extra digits on each hand, and a large mass in his chest. He was whisked to the adjoining ICU room with the neonatologist, the pastor, and Dad. Evan was quickly baptized as the neonatologist assessed him.

Sandy noticed that the new dad was very pale and diaphoretic. She guided him into a lounge chair as he began to faint.

Simultaneously the rest of the grandparents were brought into the room to see their grandson struggling to breathe. Sandy then talked with the neonatologist, took Evan from the ICU area, and placed him on his mother's chest. Evan began to coo and breathe. His breathing sounded abnormal because of the cleft in the lip and palate. It was more of a snoring, but Evan was alive and both Mom and Dad had precious time to spend with their little one.

Sandy quickly completed post-delivery care of Mom, re-set the room to a more comfortable arrangement, and assessed all the visitors in the room. She had conducted a symphony of professionals, family members, and a near-death of an infant. The music heard was the soft cooing of a baby to his parents' quiet singing.

When the daylight shift ended, neither the new nurse nor Sandy had any intention of leaving. They stayed with this family and set the postpartum care of the baby and mother in motion.

Two hours later, Sandy took the nurse grandmother aside. She explained that a different neonatologist (one that hadn't been a member of the delivery team) was going to consult with the new parents regarding what to do with their child. Evan was still alive, and decisions had to be made.

Wanting the new parents to have as much support as possible, Sandy gave the medically knowledgeable grandmother information to prepare for the meeting with the physician. With this preparation, the meeting with the physician went well.

Sandy helped transfer this new family to the postpartum floor. She arranged a room at the end of the hallway, away from the mothers with normal babies. She wished the family well and left them in capable hands. Evan passed away at 10 p.m., roughly 14 ½ hours after the couple arrived at the hospital.

At 6 a.m. the next morning, the parents heard a gentle knocking on their hospital door. Sandy peeked into the room to see the mourning parents, shortly before their discharge. She offered her condolences and congratulated them on their faith and strength to provide their baby with such love for his short life. She then said goodbye and entered the labor and delivery department to see what was on the assignment board for that day.

DEFINITION:

har•di•ness

> Hardiness is a cluster of attitudes and skills that help nurses develop both courage and strategies to turn stressful circumstances from potential calamities into growth experiences. When the day becomes stressful and the sympathetic nervous system is stimulated, hardiness allows the nurse to focus on compassionate and effective solutions rather than stress. With this focus, the nurse can call upon his or her hero resources to serve patients and their families. The nurse can also find the resilience needed to come to a stressful work environment day after day.

Sandy demonstrated this hero trait from the minute she saw her assignment of both an abnormal delivery and a new hire to orient. As each hour passed, she remained resilient and upbeat. She paid particular attention to the detailed instructions this family had given. Sandy's knowledge, experience, competence, and positive attitude provided the hardiness to care for this family effectively in spite of the many challenges during and immediately after the delivery.

TIPS FOR DEVELOPING HARDINESS

You get what you get and you don't get upset.
—*Abigail Frances Turka*

BE PATIENT WITH YOURSELF

Developing hardiness takes practice and time. If you find yourself flustered in a stressful situation, take deep breaths. Do your best to focus on solutions. Do not beat yourself up for being human. With time and patience, you will develop hardiness.

PRACTICE HABITS OF RESILIENCE

Take frequent inventories of the strengths you bring to your job and personal life.

Affirm yourself for positive contributions.

Build a strong and supportive social network.

Take time for healthy meals, especially breakfast, each day.

Practice good sleep habits to allow your body to re-set after stressful days.

Make time to exercise, relax, and rejuvenate yourself regularly. Consider walks in nature, regular trips to the gym, and/or yoga classes.

Develop your problem-solving skills.

Give yourself permission to be human and make mistakes.

As the Saying Goes, "Don't Sweat the Small Stuff"

Conserve your energy by developing flexibility around daily occurrences. When annoyed or frustrated, ask yourself, "Will this matter five years from now?" If the answer is, "No," let it go. Use your energy to find solutions for the "big stuff."

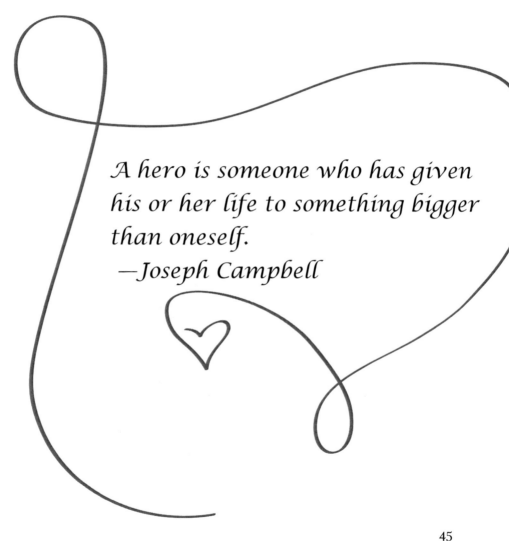

A hero is someone who has given his or her life to something bigger than oneself.
—Joseph Campbell

Give a man a fish and he will eat for a day; teach a man to fish and he will eat for a lifetime.
—**Chinese Proverb**

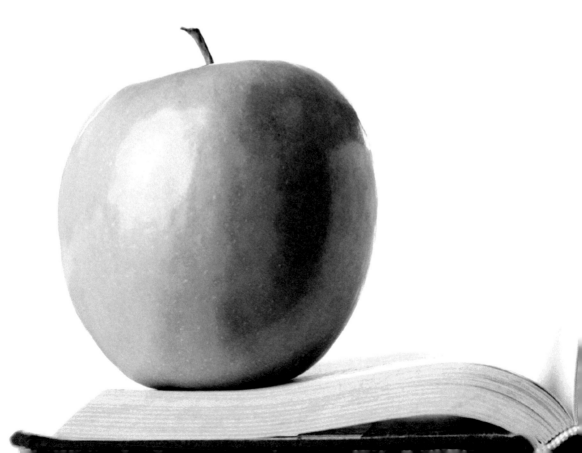

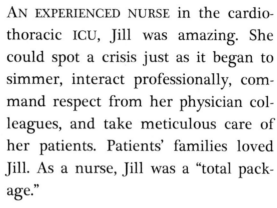

Keep Learning

An experienced nurse in the cardio-thoracic ICU, Jill was amazing. She could spot a crisis just as it began to simmer, interact professionally, command respect from her physician colleagues, and take meticulous care of her patients. Patients' families loved Jill. As a nurse, Jill was a "total package."

Jill eventually became the educator for her unit, organizing and presenting many lectures and educational vignettes. As she was becoming more involved with education, Jill was also noticing some disturbing changes in her body.

Jill noticed increasing pain and discomfort in her back and hips. A deterioration of the bone and ligament structures made it more and more difficult for her to turn and lift critically ill adults on her unit. She also had some shoulder deterioration that might require surgery.

Noticing these changes, Jill began to aspire to work in the department of education. Unfortunately, positions there required a master's degree. Jill was a graduate of a diploma program in nursing and had not continued her formal education.

Married and the mother of four children, with two still in high school, Jill made the commitment to continue her education. After 15 months of intense study, Jill completed her Bachelor of Science in Nursing (BSN). With the goal of a position in education, she immediately enrolled in and completed the Masters of Science in Nursing (MSN). This took an additional three years.

While Jill had made important contributions as a diploma graduate, she found that many more opportunities opened as she progressed through her formal college courses. Jill continues to be amazing; she can still spot a crisis while it is simmering; but now she has the skill set and credentials to teach new and inexperienced nurses how to look for subtle changes and make interventions to prevent further decline. She is also more skilled at applying the transformational leadership role of nursing as she collaborates with her medical colleagues.

DEFINITION:

learn•ing

> Every nurse must make decisions about his or her formal and informal education. The various paths into nursing licensure and varying continuing education requirements fuel all kinds of debate.
>
> What level of preparation creates the most knowledgeable, caring, compassionate, and accountable nurse? This debate has no definitive answer. No matter how you answer the question about formal education, a true commitment to patient care in a changing technical environment demands continual learning.

Hero nurses like Jill consider nursing their career and mission in life, rather than simply their job. Not all of these nurses continue on a formal degree path, but they all keep learning. They read published research articles, attend local or national conferences, and/or attend educational offerings at their job site. Jim Rohn, the entrepreneur and motivational speaker, summarized it best when he said, "Formal education will make you a living. Self-education will make you a fortune."

TIPS TO LIFELONG LEARNING

There is no end to education. It is not that you read a book, pass an examination, and finish with education. The whole of life, from the moment you are born to the moment you die, is a process of learning.
— *Jiddu Krishnamurti*

JOIN A PROFESSIONAL ORGANIZATION

Pick the organization that most interests and challenges you. You don't need to be an officer in the organization; just gather with your peers and attend education dinner meetings and conferences. Participate as much as you can. Enjoy meeting people from other organizations. Use this time to expand your network and your knowledge.

COMPLETE YOUR CERTIFICATION

Certification in a specialty in nursing is significant. It communicates professionalism and provides both you and the patient more confidence in the care you provide. Certification validates competence—to co-workers, patients, and yourself.

READ SOMETHING NEW EVERY DAY
Spend a minimum of 30 minutes each day reading. Read to enhance your leadership and management skills. Learn about a specific disease or new surgical intervention. Read beyond healthcare-related content. Share what you are reading with your co-workers and supervisors. Make reading a habit.

NETWORK WITH OTHERS
Notice that "others" is non-specific. Be open to meeting and listening to professionals from different disciplines. Carefully consider opposing viewpoints. Listen for facts and scientific support as you converse with others. You can learn a lot in chance meetings and random conversations.

NEVER SAY NEVER
Don't be too quick to say, "I am never going back to school. I will never have a DNP or PhD." Nursing as a career provides a huge sea of possibilities. Dip your toe in the water of education and see how it feels. It may entice you to take a plunge!

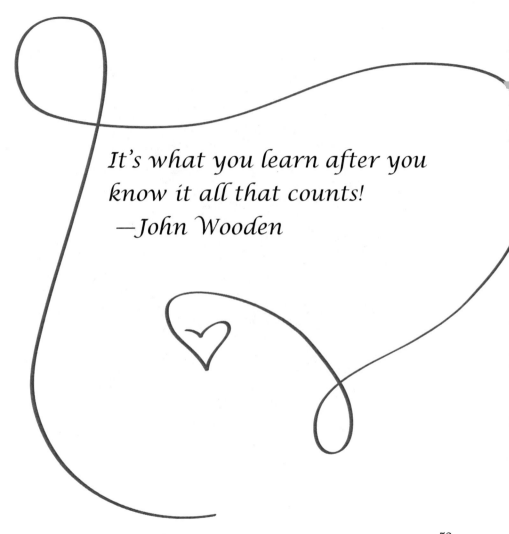

It's what you learn after you know it all that counts!
—John Wooden

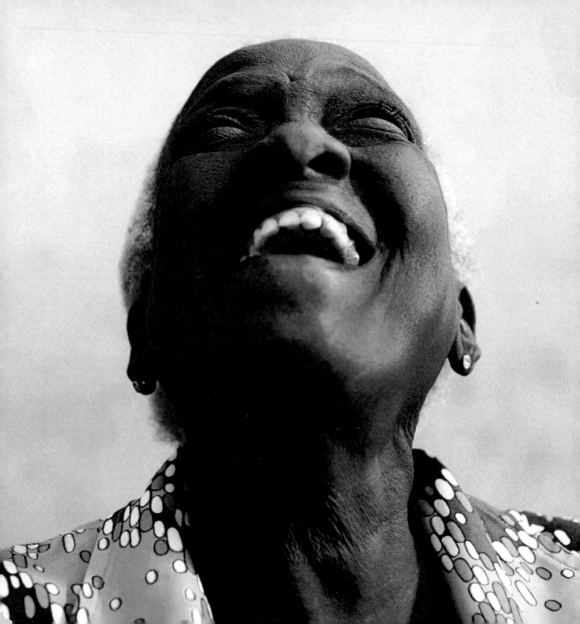

LAUGH

The human race has only one really effective weapon and that is laughter.
—Mark Twain

SOMETIMES A PATIENT SIGNALS that humor will help him or her cope with illness. For example, Mary, an oncology patient, was a "frequent flyer" to the unit. Whenever she was admitted, Mary would enter the unit by announcing, "I missed you all so much, I came back!" The staff would respond with creative and welcoming quips about the great food, scenery, or entertainment available there. The repartee between Mary and hospital staff members eased tensions on both sides and allowed Mary to cope in ways helpful to her. Mary started the laughter and humor with sarcastic remarks. Staff members followed her lead.

Another patient, Stan, had frequent blood draws to assess his chemotherapy regimen. Stan's favorite line was, "Here comes the vampire to suck my blood again." Depending on the nurse, a five-minute banter with Stan and the nurse competing for the best Bella Lugosi imitation of, "I want your blood!" would ensue. Some nurses were better at the imitation than others, but as each followed Stan's lead, laughter resounded through the halls. The childlike moments these nurses shared with Stan brightened their days. Most importantly, they gave Stan a healthy break from the job of being incredibly sick.

Norman Cousins was the first patient to publish a personal account supporting the role of laughter in healing. Without a hero doctor who took his cue from the patient, this would not have been possible.

Cousins was diagnosed with a painful, crippling, and irreversible disease. Rather than languish and die in a hospital, Cousins told his physician he wanted to go home and try an experiment. He wanted to use his own powers of faith, love, and laughter to heal himself. Against all odds, the doctor said, "Okay," and collaborated with Cousins in this unique, life-and-death adventure.

In his bestselling book, *Anatomy of an Illness,* Cousins describes how he "laughed his way out of a crippling disease." Cousins explains how 10 minutes of hardy laughing to Marx Brothers movies provided him at least 2 hours of being pain free. Cousins laughed his way through another decade-plus of life before he died in 1990. *Anatomy of an Illness*, a seminal book, is still on the market in a 20th anniversary edition. A hero physician, willing to follow one patient's desire to laugh, made this possible.

Laughter can pave the way to healthy relationships with physicians, residents, and ancillary staff as well as patients. Well-placed laughter puts everyone at ease and relaxes the generally tense atmosphere of a medical area.

Nurses, in addition, are also known to have a macabre sense of humor that can send an entire unit into fits of laughter. This humor belongs in the nursing lounge, behind closed doors and out of hearing of the patient and family. This humor breaks the tension around some of the most critical or difficult of hospital experiences. For example, "We needed waders on to clean up the code brown down the hall."

DEFINITION:

laugh

> Hero nurses use laughter as a weapon against the villains of illness, pain, and suffering. It's also a gratifying type of exercise. Muscle contraction occurs in fifteen facial muscles, the diaphragm, abdominal, shoulder, and back muscles.

Laughter results in an increase in heart rate and blood flow as well as increased respiratory excursion and increased oxygenation. This increased respiratory and cardiac workout rejuvenates the body by providing exercise to these organs and fresh oxygen-filled blood flow to every cell in the human body.

Laughter also provides a "feel good" response by releasing chemical endorphins into the bloodstream and preventing the release of cortisol and epinephrine, the stress hormones. Laughter increases the release of infection-fighting antibodies that promote a healthier immune system as well as healing.

Hero nurses know that laughter benefits the patient, both physically and emotionally. Humor is an integral part of compassionate care. Humor also helps the healthcare team manage assignments more effectively and thoughtfully. The increased oxygenation and circulation in the brain helps them to think more clearly and accurately. While saving lives and caring for the ill is serious business, hero nurses know that sensitive, respectful, and well-placed laughter is healthy for all.

Tips to Maintain a Healthy Sense of Humor

I love people who make me laugh . . . . It cures a
multitude of ills. It's probably the most important
thing in a person.
—Audrey Hepburn

Surround Yourself with Positive, Fun-Loving People
When others around you are laughing and light hearted, you absorb this upbeat experience and pass it on. Positive perspectives are contagious. If you don't have fun-loving people at work, find them in other areas of your life.

Participate in Activities that Allow You to Regain Your Childhood Sense of Wonder
Such activities may include playing games, watching funny movies, interacting with children, visiting a zoo or amusement park, etc. Whatever relaxes you and allows you to feel like a child again, is a good thing to do.

Follow Your Patient's Cues
Don't be afraid to laugh or have fun at work. It can lighten the patient's mood and provide a positive connection. Just use sensitivity and follow each patient's lead.

Do a Little Reading

Consider the following practical books on humor in healthcare:

The Healing Power of Humor by Allen Klein

Anatomy of an Illness: As Perceived by the Patient by Norman Cousins

Head First: The Biology of Hope and the Healing Power of the Human Spirit, by Norman Cousins

Carefully Guard the Macabre Humor

While this humor can break the tension productively among those in the healthcare team, it has the potential to wound patients and families. Keep it in the lounge where it belongs.

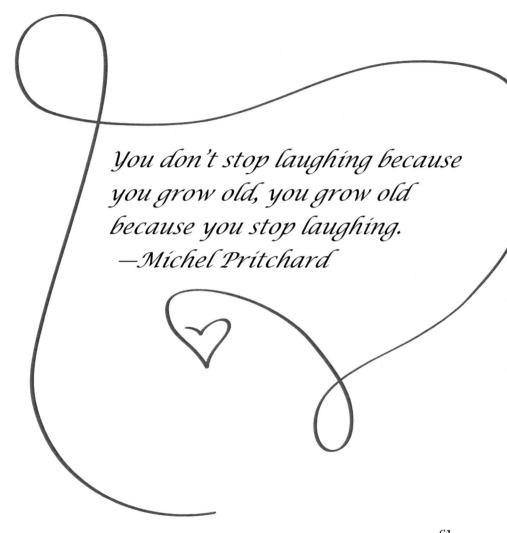

You don't stop laughing because you grow old, you grow old because you stop laughing.
—Michel Pritchard

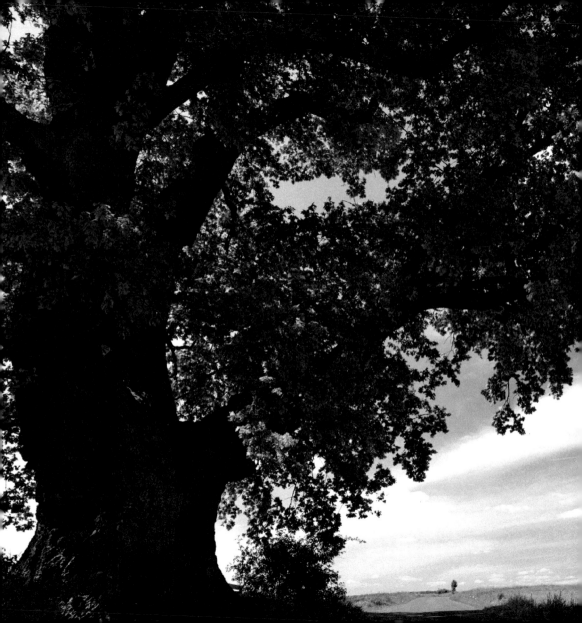

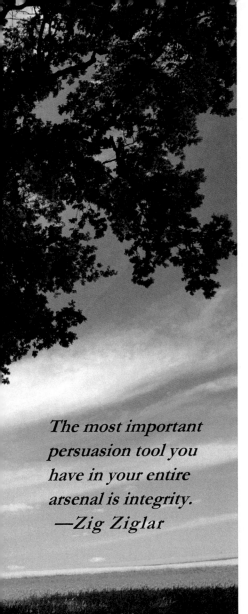

The most important persuasion tool you have in your entire arsenal is integrity.
—*Zig Ziglar*

LIVE WITH INTEGRITY

ON THE MONITORED CARDIAC UNIT THAT DAY, Linda had five patients. It seemed she couldn't catch her breath as call lights rang and monitors bonged. As she administered medications to her patients, Linda was planning to catch up. She was, of course, careful to make sure each patient had the correct blood pressure and heart rate so she could deliver the correct drug to each patient.

Linda was feeling hopeful about her progress as she entered Mr. G.'s room. A pleasant man in his 50s, Mr. G. had been admitted with a myocardial infarction that resulted in some heart failure. His salt and pepper hair fell into his face as he engaged Linda in conversation. A laborer by profession, Mr. G. was in remarkable shape for a man in his 50s. On this particular day, Mr. G. was also very talkative.

As Mr. G. continued to talk, Linda had the sinking realization that he was gearing up for a long conversation with more questions than she had time to answer. She had been expecting to simply administer the medications and return to her busy day. Not this time. Mr. G. was asking questions about the medications.

Linda explained that she was providing the same pills as the previous day and hurried to get Mr. G. to swallow. She then rushed to her next patient to do the same.

That patient said, "I have never taken this many pills before." As a precaution, Linda looked at her medication administration sheet, and she was soon overwhelmed with panic. Linda couldn't believe it: In the rush to leave Mr. G.'s room, she had given him the wrong medications.

Linda sprinted to Mr. G.'s room, completed a set of vital signs and placed a call to the cardiologist. The cardiologist was a well-known tyrant, but Linda did not focus on the doctor's response. She was terrified of the reaction Mr. G. might experience from receiving the wrong medications. She monitored him closely, completed the incident report, and discussed the situation with the cardiologist.

It never occurred to Linda to hide her mistake or make excuses. Linda knew that a rule of accountability and responsibility is clearly defined in the Code of Ethics for Nurses. While Linda followed the code, it was more because of her personal commitment to integrity than because a rule was written down.

With this mistake more than 20 years behind her, Linda is currently a member of the education department of the hospital. A daily part of her job is to review incident reports and "near misses." She also is charged with teaching new nurses about the Joint Commission National Patient Safety Goals. Delivering medications safely is patient safety goal NPSG.03.06.01. Linda knows this one by heart.

While many nurse educators would leave the story of their own medication error buried in the past, Linda shares her story as an example of what not to do. It is amazing to watch her tell the story. In the telling, the listener feels he or she is right there in Mr. G.'s hospital room. The emotion, angst, and detail of the experience are that clear. Linda relates a horrible mistake of her own to help others avoid harming their patients. That's integrity.

Definition:

in•teg•ri•ty

> In simple terms, integrity is doing the right thing in every circumstance whether someone is watching or not. It's not always easy to be honest and stick to strong moral principles in the busy healthcare environment. It's not easy to admit mistakes in life-and-death situations. It's not easy to speak up when things are not right or when a colleague or patient is mistreated. But that's just what hero nurses like Linda do.

In their yearly survey, the Gallup organization asks, "Please tell me how you would rate the honesty and ethical standards of people in these different fields—very high, high, average, low, or very low?" Since being included in the Gallup poll in 1999, nurses have received the highest ranking every year except in 2001 (the year of 9/11) when fire fighters received the top honors. Hero nurses practice integrity on a continual basis to ensure the profession deserves this honor.

Tips to Maintain Integrity

In a moment of decision, the best thing you can do is the right thing. The worst thing you can do is nothing.
—*Theodore Roosevelt*

Be Truthful in All Things

Never succumb to the temptation of a "white lie" or "stretch of the truth." Keep every interaction honest. Then you'll never have to worry about what might be uncovered about you in the future.

Surround Yourself with Honest People

People who demonstrate dishonesty in one situation, can't be trusted in any situation. If a nurse calls off ill to go Christmas shopping, that nurse might also fail to report an error. Spend your time with people of integrity. These people will serve as mentors and guides when tough situations arise.

Be a Role Model

Not everyone has been raised to live with integrity, but everyone can learn from excellent examples. Demonstrate the benefits of living a life of integrity in both your personal and professional life. You may never know the positive impact you have on others, especially new nurses who look up to you.

ADMIT YOUR MISTAKES

Linda will never forget her medication error, and she will never forget Mr. G. Both ended up doing fine. This experience has allowed Linda to share her story and be an example of integrity regarding medical mistakes for many new nurses. Linda follows in the steps of Florence Nightingale, who said, "I attribute my success to this: I never gave or took an excuse."

STAY AWAY FROM DUPLICITOUS TALK AND ACTION

Refuse to participate in any culture of backstabbing or bullying behavior. Follow this rule: If you can't say it to the person's face, don't say it at all.

WHEN SAFETY IS AT STAKE, SPEAK UP

When you see or hear behavior that threatens someone's safety or violates a person's right to respect, speak up. This may be costly behavior on your part, but it is also hero behavior and the right thing to do.

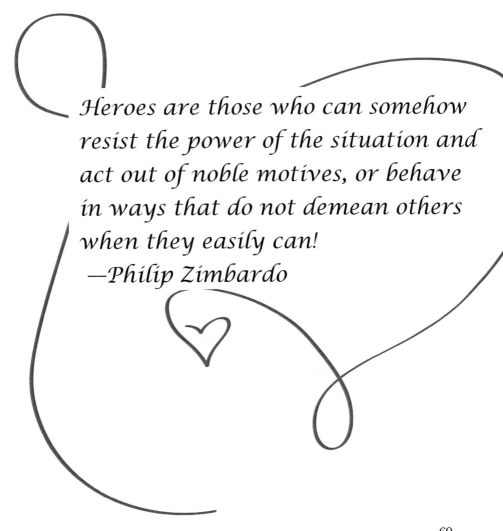

Heroes are those who can somehow resist the power of the situation and act out of noble motives, or behave in ways that do not demean others when they easily can!
—Philip Zimbardo

An attitude of positive expectation is the mark of the superior personality.
—Brian Tracy

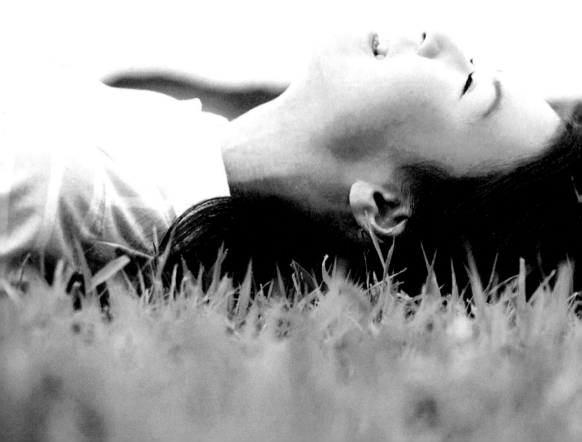

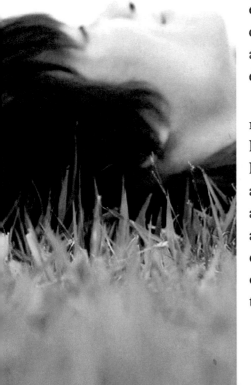

THINK POSITIVE

CHRISTINE PLACED HER HAND ON THE DOOR to the nursing department and stopped. She didn't know if she could be the happy director one more day. After all, she was supporting a number of family members in the face of tragedy. But Christine knew people were depending on her, so she paused, took a deep breath, smiled, and opened the door.

Christine works as the director of nursing education for a large tertiary hospital. To get to her office, Christine has to enter the nursing department and walk past several administrative assistants. Every day when Christine arrives at work, a show begins. She opens the door to the department, claps her hands, waves those hands in the air, and shouts, "Ta Da! I'm here!"

Anyone who is in the department, including the administrative assistants, responds by clapping and shouting, "Yay! Christine is here!"

Once Christine arrives, for the next few minutes, everyone is smiling and happy. Her upbeat perspective influences everyone's day.

Christine is well known for being the fixer, for solving problems, and for consistently displaying a positive attitude. For example, when an instructor doesn't show up to teach renal failure to a room of 100 nurses, Christine somehow manages to find someone to fill in within a matter of moments. When Christine and her 30 new nurses arrive for a nurse residency session and discover the last CPR instructor left the manikins out, Christine turns the problem into a game of "let's put the dead guys away."

Everyone who has the privilege of learning from Christine says the same thing: "She's amazing. Always has a positive attitude and is fun to be around."

However, Christine has experienced a number of family tragedies over the past few years. Her sister suddenly became acutely ill, was diagnosed with pulmonary hypertension, and needed a double lung transplant. Christine's 30 year-old son-in-law suffered an unexpected stroke. Her daughter's second child lived a mere six hours before dying in his mother's arms (with Christine by her side). There were days when Christine didn't know how she was going to make it through the day. Anyone with so many horrific personal tragedies would have a difficult time staying positive.

Every day, however, when Christine stands in front of the door to the nursing department, she puts her hand on the door-knob, takes a deep breath, and says to herself, "When I cross the threshold of my work environment, it's 'game on.' " She then turns the knob and, with a smile and a "Ta Da," starts her day.

In spite of her difficulties, Christine really is upbeat and positive. She pictures her glass as half-full. During the time when Christine's personal tragedies were at their worst, only Christine's close friends and colleagues knew the true extent of what she was going through. To the rest of the world, Christine was as upbeat as usual; people had no idea of the burdens she carried.

Of course, Christine is only human, and she struggled and grieved over the losses in her life, just as anyone would. But Christine made the choice to think positive a long time ago.

When confronted with these personal problems, Christine reached for bright moments, practical solutions, and hope for better days, just as she does on difficult days at work. Her optimism, humor, and collaborative spirit were blessings to family members and the healthcare teams who cared for them.

To those who know Christine well, it's no surprise that she puts on her game face before walking into work. They know her rah-rah spirit is more than an act—it's a choice that makes Christine a hero in every relationship, personal and professional.

DEFINITION:

pos•i•tive

Hero nurses don't spend their time complaining or waiting for someone else to improve their environments. No matter how bad the situation, these nurses take a half-full, proactive stance. They find the smile inside; they find things to appreciate in others; and they find practical solutions. The cumulative effect of positivity leads to better patient outcomes, higher patient satisfaction AND higher employee satisfaction.

Studies show that people who generally think positive have longer life spans, lower rates of depression, better psychological health, more frequent promotions, and better stress management and coping skills.

Nurses who think positive are better able to demonstrate the value they bring to the delivery of care. They influence positive thinking in others. Even nurses lacking positions of power can think positive and spread optimism—by calling on the mirror neurons in the brain.

The mirror neurons are the ones that mimic what they "see." For example, when one person in a group yawns repeatedly, others begin to do the same. Before you know it, the entire group is yawning.

Understanding the science behind this can help a nurse create a positive work environment even in the crustiest place. When one person starts a positive behavior and repeats it consistently, that behavior will spread. While positivity is not a magic pill with the power to change everything, it does make a real difference. It's an important hero behavior.

Tips to Think Positive

> *It takes but one positive thought when given a*
> *chance to survive and thrive to overpower an*
> *entire army of negative thoughts.*
> —*Robert H. Schuller*

Demonstrate Your Decision to Think Positive

Make the decision, as Christine did, that when you cross the threshold of your work environment, no matter what else is going on in your life, it's "game on." Demonstrate your choice at the beginning of each day with a smile, a word of appreciation, or a generous gesture. Avoid the temptation to begin your day whining or complaining.

Act "As If"

If you happen to tend toward a negative attitude, it's okay. You can learn to shift your brain and become more positive. Act "as if" you are genuinely happy, even if you are not. Why? Because brain science tells us that if you pretend to be happy, your brain starts to think you are and will perpetuate this. Over time, you will BE happier and so will your co-workers!

Replace Negative with Positive

Look for upbeat solutions to everyday problems. For example, one nurse worked on a unit that had the worst VRE swab scores. In response to this negative situation, the staff got together and instituted "Butt Swab Sundays." Each Sunday night, they took turns bringing in chips and salsa. But they didn't allow themselves to partake in the festivities until all of the VRE swabs were done. The staff members actually began to look forward to Sunday nights, were happier, and achieved the highest VRE compliance scores in the hospital!

Just Smile

Smiling sends happy chemical messages throughout your brain. In addition, when someone's brain "sees" a smile, it can't help but smile in return. Over time, the more you smile, the more others smile, and the happier you and they are. Never underestimate the power of a simple smile.

DO A LITTLE READING

Consider the following practical books on positivity:

Learned Optimism: How to Change Your Mind and Your Life by Martin E. P. Seligman

The Optimism Advantage: 50 Simple Truths to Transform Your Attitudes and Actions into Results by Terry L. Paulson.

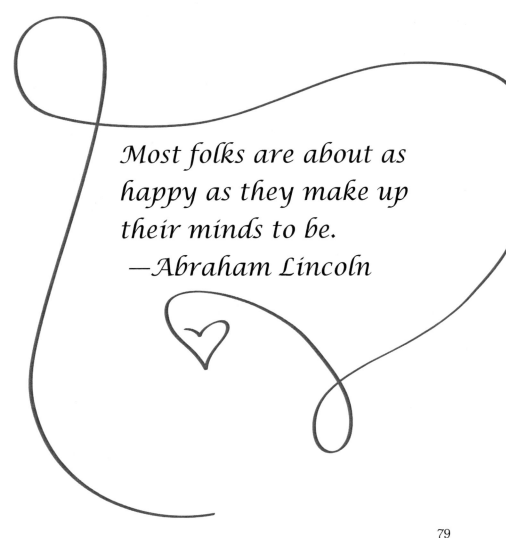

Most folks are about as happy as they make up their minds to be.
—*Abraham Lincoln*

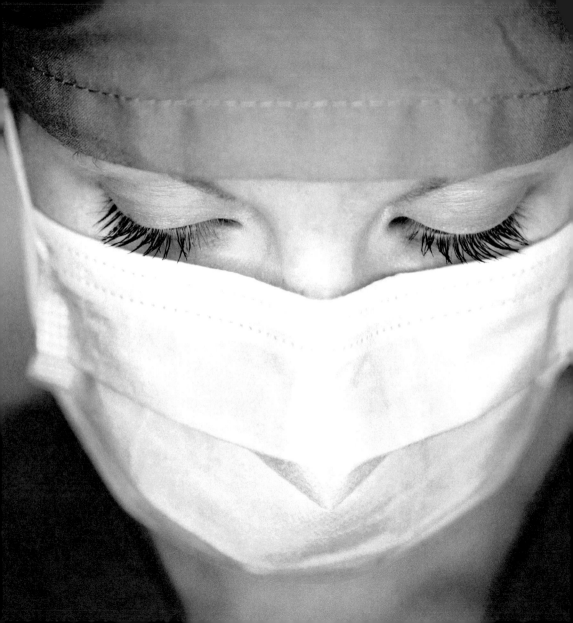

Own Your Practice

Dreams get you started; discipline keeps you going.
—Jim Rohn

SARAH WAS A SENIOR NURSING STUDENT in Rhonda's clinical group. Typically, at the beginning of a clinical rotation, students looked either scared to death or uninterested (as if they had better things to do). Sarah was different.

Sarah's uniform was clean and neatly pressed. Hair pulled away from her face, wearing minimal jewelry and make-up, Sarah was as focused as a laser on Rhonda's every word! As Rhonda spoke, Sarah was the only student taking notes.

Throughout the semester, while some students sat at the nurses' station chatting about their weekends, Sarah could always be found in either a patient's room or helping the other nurses or nursing assistants. When questioned, Sarah knew everything about her patients—even things that weren't in their charts. Why? Because when done caring for her patients, Sarah sat and talked with them.

When Sarah had a question, she asked. When the doctors rounded, Sarah was present, observing and listening. When the hospital offered an in-service, Sarah was there even if it meant returning to work after her shift. Sarah was involved in her student nurse association and frequently helped other students.

Rhonda knew Sarah was going to be an amazing nurse because Sarah took full responsibility for everything—her education, her knowledge, her skills—everything. Once, while helping her pass medications, Rhonda couldn't help herself. She told Sarah to call her parents when she returned to her dorm room. Rhonda suggested Sarah tell her parents they should be proud of her.

About a year later, Rhonda was reading an article in a school of nursing magazine about a young nurse who spent time providing care to patients in poverty-stricken areas around the world. Then Rhonda saw the picture. It was Sarah. Of course, it was Sarah. Not only had Sarah secured a great job when she graduated as a pediatric nurse, she was traveling to provide nursing care to children all over the world!

Every now and then, Rhonda still runs into Sarah. Each time, Rhonda learns more about Sarah's nursing practice and her ever-expanding role. Sarah still has the look of intention and seriousness about her practice, but now Rhonda also sees the joy of being a nurse on Sarah's face. Sarah is a hero nurse who inspires everyone around her.

DEFINITION:

own

> There is a difference between "owning" your practice and "renting" it. How do you tell the difference? The "renter" is passive, waiting for others to guide each step of the way. The "owner" is active, taking responsibility for each step of his or her own career.

Sarah demonstrated the hero behavior of owning her practice by taking every opportunity to learn, both inside and outside of her work unit. Once Sarah's formal training was behind her, she continued to own her practice, always learning and moving forward in her career and her volunteer work.

Hero nurses own their own practice and take responsibility for the role they play in the delivery of healthcare. Owning your practice means taking full responsibility for your nursing career.

Tips to Own Your Practice

Opportunity is missed by most people, because it is dressed in overalls and looks like work.
—Thomas Edison

Stay on Top of Your Own Professional Responsibilities

Nurses who take full responsibility don't wait for an e-mail to remind them it's time to renew their licenses or that their competencies are due. These nurses already know; they do what it takes to maintain their competence whether they are paid for their time or not. Owning your practice means you are aware of your responsibilities and take action on them. Remember, ignorance isn't a defense.

Be a Part of the Solution

Nurses often complain about what's wrong with healthcare—they complain about pharmacy, other nurses, administration, physicians, and even patients and their families. Just think if all the energy wasted on complaining was invested in coming up with solutions. Since 95% of all decisions happen at the point of care, nurses are in the perfect role to become problem-solvers. Own your practice by refusing to jump onto the bandwagon of complaints. Actively focus on solutions.

EXPAND YOUR SCOPE

"That's not my patient" is the worst phrase to come out of a nurse's mouth! Owning your practice means looking beyond your assignment, beyond your shift, even beyond your unit. Expand—collaborate—respect each other—own it.

GET INVOLVED

Nursing is more than a Monday-through-Friday, 9-to-5 job. It requires diligence to go beyond the hours at work to maintain and grow in your profession. Own your practice by reading journal articles related to your patient-specific population. Access the library for help. Serve on committees and participate in driving nursing practice in your organization. Hero nurses who own their practice are involved.

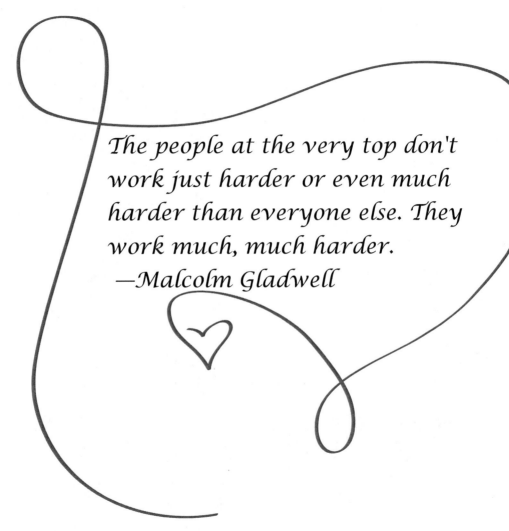

The people at the very top don't work just harder or even much harder than everyone else. They work much, much harder.

—Malcolm Gladwell

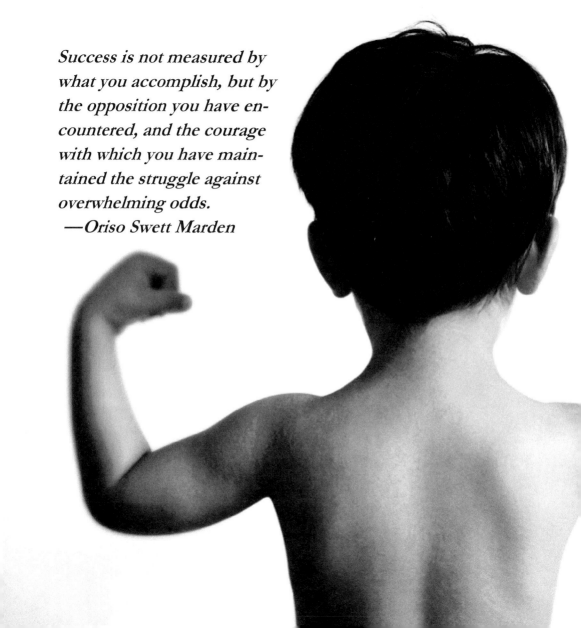

Success is not measured by what you accomplish, but by the opposition you have encountered, and the courage with which you have maintained the struggle against overwhelming odds.
—*Oriso Swett Marden*

Strengthen Moral Courage

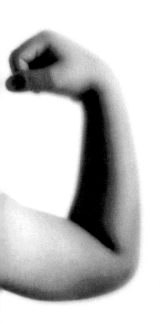

ONE LOOK AT KATIE'S FACE and Jan knew there was a problem.

Katie, a young charge nurse in a busy neurological ICU, had recently been promoted to the charge position. Jan's role as a clinical nurse specialist was to round on the intensive care units to educate nurses, review patient care, and support clinical decision-making.

Assuming there were patient problems on the unit, Jan asked Katie if she needed help. Although Katie said everything was fine, she was sweating, shaking, and looking like she was about to throw up! Jan persisted in offering help until Katie finally took a deep breath and, holding back tears, said, "Yes. I'm in a crisis situation and don't know what to do."

Here's the scenario Katie faced: Most of the nurses on the unit worked 12-hour shifts and had a patient-to-nurse ratio of 2:1. On this particular day, one of the neuro nurses had to leave at 3 p.m. Luckily, the unit was getting a float pool nurse to replace this nurse for the four-hour gap. It so happened that the nurse who was leaving would also be transferring both of her patients. That meant two open beds for the 3 p.m. to 7 p.m. float pool nurse.

Jan didn't see the problem until Katie told her the unit had two patients on its admission list. Both were fresh post-op craniotomies. Fresh post-ops are typically the most critical patients in the ICU. They require more attention, skill, and care than other patients.

As charge nurse, Katie could either assign the float pool nurse the two fresh craniotomies, or she could ask one of the existing 12-hour nurses to give up her two patients mid-shift and take the two new post-op patients. While the float pool nurse was an ICU nurse, he did not have neuro experience.

To Jan, the choice seemed obvious. Katie needed to ask one of the remaining nurses to give up her assignment to take the two fresh craniotomies. A nurse would be inconvenienced, but patients must always come first.

As Jan discussed this with Katie, the real reason for Katie's stress emerged. The only nurse whose assignment was appropriate to switch was Rita. Rita was a bully, and not just any bully. Rita was known as the "queen bully" on this unit.

Rita was an excellent neuro nurse, but she was mean and nasty to her co-workers. Everyone was afraid of Rita, even the physicians! Several nurses on the unit had quit because of Rita's bullying behavior.

When Katie was hired, Rita had referred to her as a baby nurse for the first three years. When Katie was promoted to the charge position, Rita took her aside and told Katie that being in the charge position didn't mean anything. Katie was still a baby nurse.

Now Katie was faced with the dilemma of asking Rita to give up her assignment, an assignment Rita had had for the last three days. Katie had to ask Rita to give up her easier assignment to admit two fresh craniotomy patients. Katie knew that even a nice nurse might resist such a change. Who knew what Rita would do? She was petrified. The very idea of the upcoming conversation was paralyzing.

Jan knew she needed to help Katie find the moral courage to face the bully. Jan pulled Katie into an empty room and asked her to sit down and take a few deep breaths. Then Jan asked, "If you were a fresh post-op craniotomy, who would you want caring for you? Would you want an experienced neuro nurse or a nurse who has no experience caring for neuro patients?"

Katie protested, "But Rita will freak out on me! She'll retaliate and make my life a living hell."

Jan replied, "As a nurse, you have an ethical responsibility to always make decisions based on what's best for our public, not us. No matter what might happen to you, you always have to do the right thing for patients."

Katie started to cry. She knew Jan was right. She knew she had to switch Rita's assignment but was terrified to approach her. Katie took a deep breath and walked back onto the unit.

Together, Jan and Katie approached Rita about the situation. Katie acknowledged to Rita that giving up her assignment to take two craniotomies was not in Rita's best interest but in the best interest of the patients.

As expected, Rita blew up and initially refused to give up her assignment. Katie stood strong. Both Katie and Jan reminded Rita that she had a responsibility to provide high quality care to their patients and that switching assignments was in the patients' best interests. Katie also offered to help Rita when her new patients arrived.

Although Rita was visibly angry, she switched her assignment with the float pool nurse and took the two fresh craniotomies. Once Katie recovered from her anxiety and stress, she felt strong and proud of herself. While she knew that fresh skirmishes with Rita were on the horizon, she felt a little more prepared for the next one. Katie was walking into her responsibilities rather than hiding from them. She was demonstrating the hero behavior of moral courage.

DEFINITION:

mor•al cour•age

> Moral courage is the ability to take action despite the risk of adversity. It's the ability to overcome fear and stand up for yourself and others, and to make decisions based on what's best for the team, not yourself, or any one individual. Moral courage ultimately is about doing the right thing—every time—no matter what.

It's only natural to be anxious in difficult situations, so Katie's fear of a bully didn't make her a failure. Katie ultimately showed hero behavior when she did the right thing in the face of her fear. The evening of this incident, Katie looked in the mirror and saw a person who was stronger than the one she had seen there in the morning.

It takes moral courage to sit for your certification exam or return to school after 15 years, intervene when a bully nurse is screaming at a new nurse in the hallway, or challenge a physician at 3 a.m. to get what you need for your patient. The good news is that moral courage is a skill you can build and strengthen, just like you build your bicep muscle. If you continuously push past the fear of standing up for what is right, your moral courage muscles will grow.

TIPS TO DEVELOP MORAL COURAGE

We must build dikes of courage to hold back the flood of fear.
—Martin Luther King, Jr.

Pause and Take a Deep Breath

It's easy to get caught up in the unpredictability of healthcare, the constant demands placed on nurses, and the emotional rollercoaster involved with life-and-death situations. Sometimes nurses make kneejerk decisions in response to dizzying complexities. However, taking the time to pause and breathe deeply gives you the mental space you need to formulate the best response. Ask yourself, "What are my options? What might be the possible consequences of each option? What option is the best for the patient?"

View the Situation from the Public's Eyes

Jan asked Katie the ultimate moral courage question, "If you were this patient, who would you want caring for you?" Always, always, view the situation through your patient's eyes. Ask yourself, "If I were this patient, what decision would I want my nurse to make?" Then make the decision you would want made for yourself or a loved one.

Listen to Your Gut

Nursing intuition is a powerful tool. It guides our decisions, alerts us when something is wrong, and ultimately protects patients. You've heard nurses say, "In my gut, I knew something was wrong." They may then have failed to act upon that feeling. Being a hero involves listening to your intuition. If something doesn't feel right, it probably isn't. When your intuition says something is wrong, investigate and ask for help. Engage in conversations about ethics and the right thing to do.

SPEAK UP

When faced with conflict, many nurses use silence as a strategy to get through. However, it's far better to speak up and defend your position than to stay silent and have regrets. If you think something isn't right (new medication order, assessment findings, etc.), speak up. You are the advocate for your patient's health and well-being. Even if you are afraid, push past your fear and speak up.

MAKE HEROIC DECISIONS

It takes moral courage to be a hero in the eyes of your patients. Moral courage is a choice. Ultimately, every decision you make needs to be in alignment with the ethical responsibilities you have to the public. When in doubt, think, WWHD: What Would a Hero Do? Once you have the answer, do it!

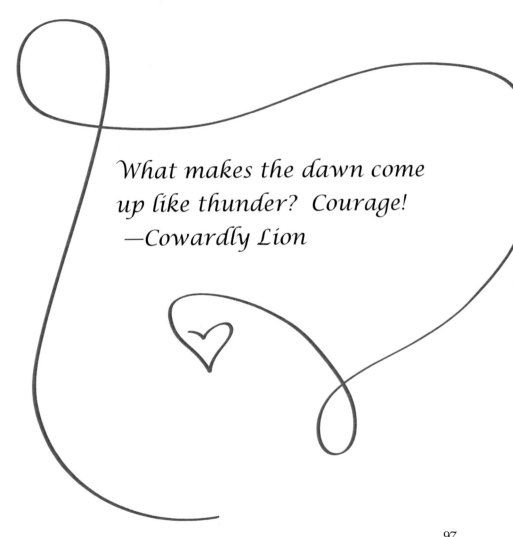

What makes the dawn come up like thunder? Courage!
—Cowardly Lion

So What, Now What?

NURSES ARE PRESENT at the moment life comes into this world and at the moment life ends. We witness incredible human strength and perseverance to survive as well as the peace displayed by humans who say "enough." We are the public's advocates, caretakers, teachers, and partners. We have an incredible opportunity to improve individual lives with compassionate care.

Of course, we all have moments when we question our decision to become nurses; when we leave work thinking it would be better just to quit and find an easier career. Although we all have days when we think we can't survive one more day, the strength inside us emerges. We somehow rise above the chaos and remember why we became nurses—to make a difference in the lives of other humans.

Every nurse performs heroic acts; it's in the nature of the job. Every nurse also has the potential to become a hero nurse—one who consistently engages in a cluster of hero behaviors that elevate patient care to an exemplary status.

As a nurse, you are born a human being; you can choose to be a hero. As you go to work in the next days, weeks, and months, step into the following cluster of behaviors:

- Extend compassion
- Communicate with openness and respect
- Build relationships
- Develop hardiness
- Keep learning
- Laugh
- Live with integrity
- Think positively
- Own your practice
- Strengthen moral courage

In choosing nursing as your profession, you've made the big choice. The path forward now consists of step-by-step, hour-by-hour behaviors that add up to heroism.

It's not easy to consistently engage in hero behaviors in the demanding environment of healthcare. Even so, you can choose to be a hero, one behavior at a time. You have a hero inside you. We're cheering as you help your hero powers grow!

ABOUT THE AUTHORS

RENEE THOMPSON, DNP, RN, CMSRN, has been a human for 40+ years and a nurse for more than 20. Several years ago, she took a leap of faith and started her own business, RTConnections. As a speaker, consultant, and coach, she is working to make a difference in the lives of nurses and the patients they serve. Renee is well known for her energizing and entertaining speaking style, along with her ability to simplify complex concepts in ways that help nurses succeed.

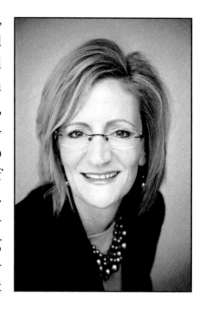

Renee speaks nationally to healthcare organizations and academic institutions, motivating audiences through keynote addresses, professional conferences, workshops, and seminars. Renee inspires nurses and other healthcare professionals in a fun and interactive fashion, sharing her vision through storytelling with meaningful life lessons and examples. Her presentations focus on improving clinical and professional competence; addressing nurse-to-nurse bullying; effective communication and leadership; embracing social media in nursing; building a positive and healthy workplace; and nurturing a culture of respect.

Renee believes that patients deserve to be cared for by competent, compassionate nurses and that nurses deserve to believe they make a difference. Because they do!

To stay connected with nurses, Renee continues to care for patients on a medical surgical step-down unit.

Renee lives in Pittsburgh, Pennsylvania with her husband Ashley.

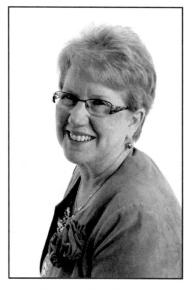

JOANNE TURKA, MSN, RN-BC, Alumnus CCRN, has over 35 years of experience in nursing, with 25+ years in critical care nursing, in both a cardiothoracic and medical/surgical ICU. On a bet, Joanne applied for a teaching position at a local university. Winning the bet, Joanne taught at the university level for 9 years, including clinical medical surgical nursing and didactic in leadership courses.

Currently, Joanne works in staff development for UPMC Shadyside. She coordinates and teaches the critical care course content, organizes and welcomes nurses in orientation, and runs the Nurse Residency Program. She is responsible for all formal education and is part of the team that reviews the policy and procedures designed to provide patient safety.

Having presented at the National Teaching Institute of the American Association of Critical Care Nurses, the Association of Medical Surgical Nurses, and the Association of Nursing

Professional Development, Joanne is an experienced speaker. She engages audiences in topics including social media, traumatic brain injury, hemodynamics for the bedside nurse, effective communication strategies, and critical care certification.

Joanne believes that nurses can only make a difference if they have the educational tools needed to do so. She is always looking for the most appropriate interactive methods to engage and teach new nurses. Joanne is known for her sense of humor and ability to teach at both very simple and complex levels. She can weave a story into a dramatic learning event and have students remember the content for decades.

Joanne lives in Pittsburgh, Pennsylvania with her husband, Donald. She is proud of her three adult children and four darling grandchildren.

Finally! A Solution to Nurse-to-Nurse Bullying

Ask any nurse if he or she has heard the phrase, "Nurses eat their young," and you'll get nods of sad recognition. Nurses choose their profession to deliver compassionate and effective patient care, and then they discover the ugly in nursing: nurses can be horrific to each other. Finally, here is a book to guide nurses along a new path.

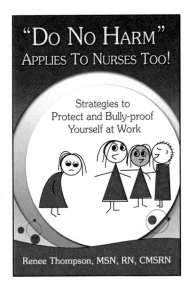

"Do No Harm" Applies To Nurses Too!

Strategies to Protect and Bully-proof Yourself at Work

Renee Thompson, MSN, RN, CMSRN

You'll learn:

- What to do to make yourself less attractive to bullies

- Specific manageable steps to stop the bullying

- Sample responses to common bully attacks in nursing

Book Renee Thompson for Your Next Event

Bring Renee to your healthcare organization or academic institution to provide solutions for the issues nurses and nursing students face today. Renee delivers keynote presentations and onsite workshops customized to meet your needs and those of your target audience: nursing leadership, faculty, educators, staff/student nurses, new nurses, and healthcare team members.

Here are a few sample presentations and programs to consider:

KEYNOTES:

- Celebrate Nursing: Human by Birth—Hero by Choice
- Navigating the Road to Exemplary Practice

WORKSHOPS:

- Communication, Conflict, and Co-workers—Oh My!
  Navigating the Yellow-Brick Road to Effective Communication

- "Do No Harm" Applies to Nurses Too!
  Strategies to Protect and Bully-Proof Yourself at Work

- Navigating the Social Media Super Highway
  Strategies for Nurse Leaders

To learn more, contact Renee at www.RTConnections.com